DR. BARBARA 7-DAY JUICING FOR CANCER CURE

Discover dr Barbara's potent remedies and transformative recipes for healing cancer naturally using nutrient packed delicious blends

Edwardo Pedro

Table of Contents

COPYRIGHT © 2023

CHAPTER ONE

Introduction to Dr. Barbara's Herbal Juicing Protocol for Cancer Healing

Dr. Barbara's Herbal Juicing Protocol for Cancer Healing is a holistic approach to complement conventional cancer treatments, focusing on the utilization of herbal juices to support the body's natural healing mechanisms. Developed by Dr. Barbara, a renowned naturopathic doctor specializing in integrative oncology, this protocol integrates the principles of herbal medicine with the latest scientific research to create a comprehensive regimen aimed at enhancing the overall well-being of cancer patients.

Understanding Cancer: A Brief Overview

Before delving into Dr. Barbara's Herbal Juicing Protocol, it's essential to grasp the basics of cancer. Cancer is a complex disease characterized by the uncontrolled growth and spread of abnormal cells in the body. These abnormal cells can form tumors and interfere with the normal functioning of organs and tissues. While the exact causes of cancer are still being researched, various factors such as genetic predisposition, environmental toxins, lifestyle choices, and immune system dysfunction can contribute to its development.

Conventional Cancer Treatments and Their Limitations

Conventional cancer treatments typically include surgery, chemotherapy, radiation therapy, targeted therapy, and immunotherapy. While these treatments have made significant strides in improving cancer outcomes and survival rates, they often come with a range of side effects and limitations. Chemotherapy and radiation therapy, for example, can cause severe nausea, fatigue, hair loss, and damage to healthy cells and tissues. Additionally, some cancer types may become resistant to standard treatments over time, necessitating alternative approaches to enhance their effectiveness.

The Role of Herbal Medicine in Cancer Care

Herbal medicine, also known as botanical medicine or phytotherapy, has been used for centuries in various cultures to promote health and treat a wide range of ailments, including cancer. Herbs contain a myriad of bioactive compounds such as polyphenols, alkaloids, flavonoids, and terpenes, which exhibit antioxidant, anti-inflammatory, immunomodulatory, and anti-cancer properties. Research has shown that certain herbs can inhibit tumor growth, enhance the body's immune response, and mitigate the side effects of conventional cancer treatments.

Dr. Barbara's Approach to Herbal Juicing

Dr. Barbara's Herbal Juicing Protocol is rooted in the belief that nature provides powerful healing tools that, when combined synergistically, can support the body in its fight against cancer. The protocol emphasizes the consumption of fresh, organic fruits, vegetables, and herbs in the form of therapeutic juices. These juices are carefully crafted to deliver a potent dose of nutrients, antioxidants, and phytochemicals directly into the body, bypassing the digestive system and providing rapid absorption and assimilation.

Key Components of Dr. Barbara's Herbal Juicing Protocol

1. **Selection of Herbal Ingredients**: Dr. Barbara's protocol incorporates a diverse array of herbs known for their anti-cancer properties, such as turmeric, ginger, garlic, green tea, astragalus, and milk thistle. Each herb is chosen for its specific therapeutic effects, including immune modulation, inflammation reduction, detoxification support, and tumor inhibition.

2. **Juicing Techniques**: To maximize the therapeutic benefits of herbal juices, Dr. Barbara recommends using a high-quality juicer to extract the maximum amount of nutrients from fresh produce. Organic fruits and vegetables should be washed thoroughly to remove any pesticides or

contaminants before juicing. It's also important to consume the juices immediately after preparation to preserve their nutritional integrity.

3. **Individualized Treatment Plans**: Dr. Barbara tailors her Herbal Juicing Protocol to the unique needs and preferences of each patient, taking into account factors such as cancer type, stage, overall health status, and dietary restrictions. Patients may be advised to incorporate specific herbs or combinations of herbs into their juicing regimen based on their therapeutic goals and tolerance levels.

4. **Integration with Conventional Therapies**: While herbal juicing is a key component of Dr. Barbara's protocol, it is designed to complement rather than replace conventional cancer treatments. Patients are encouraged to continue their prescribed treatments under the guidance of their oncologists while incorporating herbal juices as a supportive adjunct therapy. This integrative approach aims to optimize treatment outcomes while minimizing side effects and improving quality of life.

Scientific Evidence Supporting Herbal Juicing for Cancer Healing

Although the scientific evidence supporting the efficacy of herbal juicing specifically for cancer healing is still evolving, numerous studies have demonstrated the anti-cancer properties of individual herbs and botanical compounds. For example, curcumin, the active ingredient in turmeric, has been shown to inhibit tumor growth, induce apoptosis (cell death) in cancer cells, and enhance the effectiveness of chemotherapy and radiation therapy. Similarly, compounds found in ginger, garlic, green tea, and other herbs have exhibited anti-inflammatory, antioxidant, and anti-cancer effects in preclinical and clinical studies.

Patient Testimonials and Clinical Outcomes

While anecdotal evidence and patient testimonials provide valuable insights into the potential benefits of Dr. Barbara's Herbal Juicing Protocol, rigorous clinical research is needed to validate its efficacy and safety in cancer patients. However, many individuals who have followed the protocol report improvements in energy levels, immune function, digestive health, and overall well-being. Some patients have also experienced reductions in tumor size, tumor markers, and cancer-related symptoms, although these outcomes may vary depending on individual factors and disease characteristics.

Conclusion

In conclusion, Dr. Barbara's Herbal Juicing Protocol for Cancer Healing offers a holistic and integrative approach to supporting the health and well-being of cancer patients. By harnessing the therapeutic power of herbs and botanicals, this protocol aims to enhance the body's natural defenses, reduce inflammation, detoxify the system, and inhibit tumor growth. While further research is needed to fully elucidate the mechanisms of action and clinical efficacy of herbal juicing in cancer care, preliminary evidence suggests that it holds promise as a complementary therapy alongside conventional treatments. Ultimately, the goal of Dr. Barbara's protocol is to empower patients to take an active role in their healing journey and optimize their chances of long-term survival and recovery.

CHAPTER TWO

The Healing Power of Herbal Juices: Understanding Their Role in Cancer Treatment

Herbal juices have long been recognized for their potential therapeutic benefits, including their role in supporting cancer treatment. In recent years, there has been a growing interest in exploring the healing properties of herbs and botanicals, particularly in the context of integrative oncology. This article aims to delve into the science behind herbal juices and their potential role in cancer treatment, exploring their mechanisms of action, evidence-based benefits, and practical considerations.

Understanding Herbal Juices: A Primer

Herbal juices are liquid extracts derived from fresh or dried herbs, fruits, and vegetables. These juices can be obtained using various methods, including juicing, blending, and decoction. Unlike commercial fruit juices, which may contain added sugars and preservatives, herbal juices are typically prepared using organic ingredients and consumed in their natural state to maximize their therapeutic potential.

Mechanisms of Action in Cancer Treatment

Herbal juices exert their anti-cancer effects through a multitude of mechanisms, targeting various pathways involved in tumor initiation, growth, and metastasis. Some of the key mechanisms of action include:

1. **Antioxidant Activity**: Many herbs contain bioactive compounds such as polyphenols, flavonoids, and carotenoids, which possess potent antioxidant properties. These antioxidants help neutralize harmful free radicals, thereby reducing oxidative stress and DNA damage, which are implicated in cancer development.

2. **Anti-inflammatory Effects**: Chronic inflammation plays a crucial role in the development and progression of cancer. Certain herbs, such as turmeric, ginger, and green tea, exhibit anti-inflammatory properties by inhibiting pro-inflammatory cytokines and enzymes, thereby modulating the inflammatory response and creating an unfavorable environment for tumor growth.

3. **Immune Modulation**: Herbal juices can enhance the body's immune response to cancer by stimulating the activity of immune cells such as T cells, natural killer cells, and macrophages. Ingredients like astragalus, echinacea, and reishi mushroom have been shown to boost immune function and improve the body's ability to identify and eliminate cancerous cells.

4. **Apoptosis Induction**: Apoptosis, or programmed cell death, is a natural process that eliminates damaged or abnormal

cells from the body. Herbal compounds like curcumin, resveratrol, and quercetin can induce apoptosis in cancer cells, preventing their uncontrolled proliferation and promoting their elimination by the immune system.

5. **Angiogenesis Inhibition**: Tumor growth and metastasis depend on the formation of new blood vessels to supply oxygen and nutrients to cancer cells. Certain herbs contain anti-angiogenic compounds that inhibit the formation of blood vessels, thereby starving tumors of their blood supply and impeding their growth and spread.

Evidence-Based Benefits of Herbal Juices in Cancer Treatment

While the scientific evidence supporting the efficacy of herbal juices in cancer treatment is still evolving, several studies have provided insights into their potential benefits:

1. **Turmeric**: Curcumin, the active compound in turmeric, has been extensively studied for its anti-cancer properties. Research suggests that curcumin can inhibit the growth of various cancer types, including breast, prostate, colon, and pancreatic cancer, by modulating multiple signaling pathways involved in tumor progression.

2. **Ginger**: Ginger contains bioactive compounds such as gingerol and shogaol, which exhibit anti-inflammatory and

anti-cancer effects. Studies have shown that ginger extract can suppress the growth and metastasis of cancer cells, induce apoptosis, and enhance the efficacy of chemotherapy and radiation therapy in preclinical models.

3. **Green Tea**: Epigallocatechin gallate (EGCG), the primary polyphenol in green tea, has been studied for its anti-cancer properties. EGCG has been shown to inhibit tumor growth, angiogenesis, and metastasis in various cancer types, including breast, prostate, lung, and colorectal cancer, through its antioxidant, anti-inflammatory, and anti-angiogenic effects.

4. **Wheatgrass**: Wheatgrass juice is rich in chlorophyll, vitamins, minerals, and enzymes, which have been attributed to its potential anti-cancer effects. Some studies suggest that wheatgrass juice can inhibit tumor growth, enhance immune function, and alleviate chemotherapy-induced side effects in cancer patients.

5. **Garlic**: Garlic contains sulfur compounds such as allicin, which possess anti-cancer properties. Research has shown that garlic extract can inhibit the growth of cancer cells, induce apoptosis, and enhance the efficacy of chemotherapy drugs in preclinical studies.

Practical Considerations for Herbal Juicing in Cancer Treatment

When incorporating herbal juices into cancer treatment, it's essential to consider the following practical considerations:

1. **Quality and Safety**: Choose organic, pesticide-free herbs and vegetables whenever possible to minimize exposure to harmful chemicals. Ensure proper hygiene and sanitation practices during juicing to reduce the risk of contamination.

2. **Individualized Approach**: Tailor the selection of herbs and ingredients based on the patient's specific cancer type, stage, treatment regimen, and overall health status. Consult with a qualified healthcare professional, such as a naturopathic doctor or integrative oncologist, to develop a personalized juicing protocol.

3. **Integration with Conventional Treatment**: Herbal juices should be used as a complementary therapy alongside conventional cancer treatments, not as a replacement. Inform the patient's oncologist about any herbal supplements or juices being consumed to avoid potential interactions or contraindications with prescribed medications.

4. **Monitoring and Evaluation**: Regular monitoring of the patient's progress and response to herbal juicing is essential

to assess its efficacy and safety. Adjust the juicing protocol as needed based on changes in the patient's condition, treatment goals, and tolerance levels.

Conclusion

In conclusion, herbal juices offer a promising adjunctive therapy in cancer treatment, harnessing the healing power of nature to support the body's innate ability to fight cancer. By targeting multiple pathways involved in tumor growth and progression, herbal juices have the potential to enhance the efficacy of conventional treatments, mitigate side effects, and improve overall quality of life for cancer patients. However, further research is needed to elucidate the optimal formulations, dosages, and safety profiles of herbal juices in various cancer types and patient populations. Through a personalized and integrative approach, herbal juicing can serve as a valuable tool in the holistic care of cancer patients, empowering them to take an active role in their healing journey.

CHAPTER THREE

Selecting the Right Herbs: Key Ingredients for Dr. Barbara's Cancer Cure Juices

In Dr. Barbara's Cancer Cure Juices, the selection of herbs is paramount, as each herb contributes unique therapeutic properties aimed at supporting the body's natural healing processes and combating cancer. Dr. Barbara's approach involves carefully selecting herbs known for their anti-cancer effects, immune-boosting properties, and overall health benefits. Below are some key ingredients commonly used in Dr. Barbara's Cancer Cure Juices, along with their respective roles and evidence-based benefits:

Turmeric (Curcuma longa)

Turmeric is perhaps one of the most extensively studied herbs for its anti-cancer properties. The active compound in turmeric, curcumin, has been shown to exhibit anti-inflammatory, antioxidant, and anti-cancer effects. Curcumin has the ability to inhibit tumor growth, induce apoptosis (cell death) in cancer cells, and suppress the proliferation of cancer stem cells. Additionally, curcumin can enhance the efficacy of conventional cancer treatments such as chemotherapy and radiation therapy, while mitigating their side effects.

Ginger (Zingiber officinale)

Ginger is another potent herb with anti-cancer properties. Ginger contains bioactive compounds such as gingerol and shogaol, which possess antioxidant and anti-inflammatory effects. Studies have shown that ginger extract can inhibit the growth and spread of cancer cells, induce apoptosis, and enhance the effectiveness of chemotherapy and radiation therapy. Additionally, ginger has been found to alleviate nausea and vomiting associated with cancer treatments, making it a valuable adjunctive therapy for cancer patients.

Green Tea (Camellia sinensis)

Green tea is rich in polyphenols, particularly epigallocatechin gallate (EGCG), which have been extensively studied for their anti-cancer effects. EGCG exhibits antioxidant, anti-inflammatory, and anti-angiogenic properties, making it a promising agent for cancer prevention and treatment. Green tea consumption has been associated with a reduced risk of various cancer types, including breast, prostate, lung, and colorectal cancer. Additionally, green tea has been shown to inhibit tumor growth, metastasis, and angiogenesis, while promoting apoptosis in cancer cells.

Garlic (Allium sativum)

Garlic is renowned for its potent anti-cancer properties, attributed to its high content of sulfur compounds such as allicin. Studies have demonstrated that garlic extract can inhibit the growth of cancer cells, induce apoptosis, and suppress tumor progression in various cancer types, including breast, colon, prostate, and stomach cancer. Garlic also exhibits antioxidant and immune-modulating effects, making it a valuable addition to cancer-fighting juices.

Astragalus (Astragalus membranaceus)

Astragalus is a traditional Chinese herb known for its immune-boosting properties. Astragalus contains polysaccharides and flavonoids that enhance immune function, stimulate the production of white blood cells, and increase the body's resistance to infections and diseases. In cancer patients, astragalus has been shown to improve immune function, reduce chemotherapy-induced side effects, and enhance overall quality of life. By supporting immune health, astragalus plays a crucial role in helping the body defend against cancer and other illnesses.

Milk Thistle (Silybum marianum)

Milk thistle is a well-known herb for liver health and detoxification. The active compound in milk thistle, silymarin, exhibits antioxidant and anti-inflammatory effects, protecting the liver from damage caused by toxins, medications, and environmental pollutants. In cancer patients undergoing chemotherapy, milk thistle supplementation has been shown to reduce liver toxicity and improve liver function tests. Additionally, milk thistle may have direct anti-cancer effects by inhibiting tumor growth and promoting apoptosis in cancer cells.

Conclusion

The selection of herbs in Dr. Barbara's Cancer Cure Juices is based on their potent anti-cancer effects, immune-boosting properties, and overall health benefits. By incorporating key ingredients such as turmeric, ginger, green tea, garlic, astragalus, and milk thistle, Dr. Barbara's protocol aims to provide comprehensive support for cancer patients, enhancing the body's natural defenses and optimizing treatment outcomes. While further research is needed to elucidate the mechanisms of action and clinical efficacy of these herbs in cancer care, preliminary evidence suggests that they hold promise as valuable adjunctive therapies in the holistic management of cancer.

CHAPTER FOUR

Crafting Healing Blends: Recipes for Dr. Barbara's Cancer-Fighting Juices

Dr. Barbara's Cancer-Fighting Juices are carefully crafted blends of fresh, organic fruits, vegetables, and herbs designed to support the body's natural healing processes and combat cancer. These recipes incorporate key ingredients known for their anti-cancer properties, immune-boosting effects, and overall health benefits. Below are some delicious and nutritious recipes inspired by Dr. Barbara's protocol:

1. Golden Glow Juice

Ingredients:

- 2 medium carrots
- 1 medium apple
- 1-inch piece of fresh ginger
- ½ teaspoon of ground turmeric
- Juice of ½ lemon

Instructions:

1. Wash the carrots, apple, and ginger thoroughly.

2. Cut the carrots and apple into smaller pieces, removing any seeds or stems.

3. Peel the ginger and cut it into smaller pieces.

4. Place the carrots, apple, ginger, and turmeric in a high-quality juicer.

5. Juice the ingredients until smooth and well combined.

6. Squeeze the lemon juice into the juice and stir gently.

7. Pour the juice into a glass and enjoy immediately.

2. Green Goddess Elixir

Ingredients:

- 1 cucumber

- 2 cups of spinach

- 1 green apple

- ½ cup of fresh parsley

- Juice of 1 lime

Instructions:

1. Wash the cucumber, spinach, apple, and parsley thoroughly.

2. Cut the cucumber and apple into smaller pieces, removing any seeds or stems.

3. Place the cucumber, spinach, apple, and parsley in a high-quality juicer.

4. Juice the ingredients until smooth and well combined.

5. Squeeze the lime juice into the juice and stir gently.

6. Pour the juice into a glass and enjoy immediately.

3. Immune-Boosting Citrus Blend

Ingredients:

- 2 oranges

- 1 grapefruit

- 1-inch piece of fresh turmeric

- ½ teaspoon of ground cinnamon

- 1 tablespoon of honey (optional)

Instructions:

1. Peel the oranges and grapefruit, removing any seeds.

2. Cut the oranges and grapefruit into smaller pieces.

3. Peel the turmeric and cut it into smaller pieces.

4. Place the oranges, grapefruit, turmeric, and cinnamon in a high-quality juicer.

5. Juice the ingredients until smooth and well combined.

6. Add honey if desired for sweetness and stir gently.

7. Pour the juice into a glass and enjoy immediately.

4. Berry Bliss Antioxidant Juice

Ingredients:

- 1 cup of mixed berries (such as strawberries, blueberries, raspberries)
- 1 kiwi
- 1 tablespoon of fresh mint leaves
- ½ teaspoon of ground flaxseeds
- 1 tablespoon of honey (optional)

Instructions:

1. Wash the berries and kiwi thoroughly.
2. Remove the stems from the strawberries and any tough ends from the kiwi.
3. Cut the kiwi into smaller pieces.
4. Place the berries, kiwi, mint leaves, and flaxseeds in a high-quality juicer.
5. Juice the ingredients until smooth and well combined.
6. Add honey if desired for sweetness and stir gently.

7. Pour the juice into a glass and enjoy immediately.

5. Healing Herbal Detox Juice

Ingredients:

- 2 celery stalks

- 1 cucumber

- 1 green apple

- 1-inch piece of fresh ginger

- 1 tablespoon of fresh cilantro leaves

- Juice of 1 lemon

Instructions:

1. Wash the celery, cucumber, apple, ginger, and cilantro thoroughly.

2. Cut the celery, cucumber, and apple into smaller pieces, removing any seeds or stems.

3. Peel the ginger and cut it into smaller pieces.

4. Place the celery, cucumber, apple, ginger, and cilantro in a high-quality juicer.

5. Juice the ingredients until smooth and well combined.

6. Squeeze the lemon juice into the juice and stir gently.

7. Pour the juice into a glass and enjoy immediately.

Conclusion

Dr. Barbara's Cancer-Fighting Juices are not only delicious but also packed with potent anti-cancer ingredients and immune-boosting nutrients. By incorporating these healing blends into your daily routine, you can support your body's natural defenses, promote overall health and well-being, and enhance your resilience in the fight against cancer. Experiment with different combinations of fruits, vegetables, and herbs to discover your favorite flavors and reap the benefits of nature's healing power.

CHAPTER FIVE

The 7-Day Juicing Plan: A Comprehensive Guide to Jumpstarting Your Healing Journey

Embarking on a 7-day juicing plan can be a transformative experience for your health and well-being, especially when tailored to support your healing journey. Whether you're seeking to boost your immune system, detoxify your body, or complement your cancer treatment regimen, a well-designed juicing plan can provide the nourishment and support your body needs to thrive. This comprehensive guide will walk you through the steps of creating and implementing a 7-day juicing plan tailored to your specific health goals.

Day 1: Preparation and Planning

Before diving into your juicing journey, take some time to prepare and plan for the week ahead:

1. **Set Your Intentions**: Clarify your health goals and intentions for the juicing plan. Whether you're aiming to detoxify, boost your energy, or support your cancer treatment, having a clear purpose will guide your choices throughout the week.

2. **Gather Your Supplies**: Ensure you have all the necessary supplies on hand, including a high-quality juicer, fresh organic produce, and storage containers for your juices.

3. **Create a Shopping List**: Plan your juicing recipes for the week and create a shopping list of the fruits, vegetables, and herbs you'll need. Aim for a diverse range of ingredients to maximize nutritional benefits.

4. **Prepare Your Workspace**: Set up your juicing station in a clean, well-lit area of your kitchen. Wash and prep your produce, and organize your ingredients for easy access.

Day 2-6: Daily Juicing Routine

Follow this daily juicing routine to nourish your body and support your healing journey:

1. **Morning Ritual**: Start each day with a glass of warm water with lemon to hydrate and alkalize your body. Follow this with a freshly prepared juice for breakfast.

2. **Mid-Morning Snack**: Enjoy a light snack, such as fresh fruit or nuts, to keep your energy levels stable until lunchtime.

3. **Lunchtime Boost**: Have another juice for lunch, focusing on ingredients that provide sustained energy and nourishment. Consider adding leafy greens, citrus fruits, and herbs for a refreshing blend.

4. **Afternoon Pick-Me-Up**: Beat the afternoon slump with a revitalizing juice or smoothie packed with nutrient-dense ingredients like kale, spinach, berries, and protein-rich seeds or nuts.

5. **Dinner Delight**: Conclude your day with a satisfying juice or smoothie that aids digestion and promotes relaxation. Consider incorporating ingredients like cucumber, celery, ginger, and mint for a refreshing evening blend.

6. **Hydration Hygiene**: Stay hydrated throughout the day by drinking plenty of water between juices to support detoxification and ensure optimal cellular function.

Day 7: Reflection and Integration

As you reach the final day of your juicing plan, take time to reflect on your experience and integrate your learnings into your daily routine:

1. **Reflect on Your Progress**: Take stock of how you feel physically, mentally, and emotionally after completing the 7-day juicing plan. Notice any changes in energy levels, digestion, mood, and overall well-being.

2. **Celebrate Your Achievements**: Acknowledge yourself for committing to your health and taking proactive steps toward healing and self-care.

3. **Transition Mindfully**: Gradually reintroduce solid foods into your diet, starting with light, easily digestible meals such as salads, soups, and steamed vegetables. Pay attention to how your body responds to different foods and make adjustments as needed.

4. **Establish Sustainable Habits**: Identify habits and practices from the juicing plan that you'd like to incorporate into your daily life moving forward. Whether it's drinking more water, consuming more fruits and vegetables, or practicing mindful eating, prioritize habits that support your long-term health and well-being.

5. **Stay Connected**: Stay connected with your body's needs and continue to nourish yourself with nutrient-rich foods, regular physical activity, restful sleep, and stress management techniques. Consider incorporating juicing into your weekly routine as a supplemental tool for ongoing health maintenance.

Conclusion

Embarking on a 7-day juicing plan is an empowering step toward enhancing your health, vitality, and resilience. By following this comprehensive guide, you can create a nourishing and supportive juicing routine that aligns with your specific health goals and needs. Whether you're seeking to detoxify, boost your immune system, or support your healing journey, juicing offers a powerful way to flood your body with essential nutrients, promote detoxification, and rejuvenate your overall well-being. Commit to your health and embrace the transformative potential of juicing as you embark on this 7-day journey toward greater health and vitality.

CHAPTER SIX

Detoxification and Renewal: How Herbal Juicing Supports the Body's Cleansing Processes

Detoxification is a natural process through which the body eliminates toxins and waste products to maintain optimal health and well-being. Herbal juicing plays a vital role in supporting the body's detoxification processes by providing a concentrated source of nutrients, antioxidants, and phytochemicals that promote cellular cleansing, rejuvenation, and renewal. This article explores the mechanisms by which herbal juicing supports detoxification and renewal, highlighting key ingredients and their benefits.

Understanding Detoxification

Detoxification is a complex physiological process that occurs primarily in the liver, kidneys, lungs, skin, and gastrointestinal tract. These organs work synergistically to neutralize and eliminate toxins, metabolic by-products, environmental pollutants, and excess hormones from the body. The liver, in particular, plays a central role in detoxification by metabolizing toxins into less harmful substances that can be excreted through urine, bile, sweat, and breath.

Role of Herbal Juicing in Detoxification

Herbal juicing provides a potent means of supporting the body's detoxification processes through several mechanisms:

1. **Nutrient Density**: Fresh fruits, vegetables, and herbs used in herbal juices are rich in vitamins, minerals, enzymes, and phytonutrients essential for optimal detoxification. These nutrients support the liver's detoxification pathways, enhance cellular repair and regeneration, and strengthen the body's defenses against oxidative stress and inflammation.

2. **Hydration**: Juicing helps maintain optimal hydration levels, which are essential for efficient detoxification. Adequate hydration supports kidney function, promotes urine production, and flushes out toxins and waste products from the body. Herbal juices provide a hydrating and nourishing alternative to sugary or caffeinated beverages that may hinder detoxification.

3. **Antioxidant Support**: Many herbs and botanicals used in herbal juices are rich in antioxidants, which help neutralize free radicals and oxidative stress. Free radicals are unstable molecules that can damage cells and tissues, contributing to aging, inflammation, and chronic disease. By scavenging free radicals, antioxidants protect cellular integrity and support overall detoxification and renewal.

4. **Liver Support**: Certain herbs, such as milk thistle, dandelion root, and burdock root, are known for their liver-protective and detoxifying properties. These herbs enhance liver function, promote bile production, and support the elimination of toxins from the body. Incorporating liver-supportive herbs into herbal juices can optimize the body's natural detoxification mechanisms and promote overall liver health.

5. **Gut Health**: Herbal juices rich in fiber, prebiotics, and digestive enzymes support gut health and bowel regularity, facilitating the elimination of toxins and waste products from the body. Fiber-rich ingredients like fruits, vegetables, and flaxseeds promote bowel movements, bind to toxins, and support the growth of beneficial gut bacteria, enhancing overall detoxification and renewal.

Key Ingredients for Detoxification and Renewal

Several key ingredients are commonly used in herbal juices to support detoxification and renewal:

1. **Dandelion Root**: Dandelion root is prized for its liver-detoxifying properties and ability to stimulate bile production, aiding in the elimination of toxins and waste products from the body.

2. **Milk Thistle**: Milk thistle contains the active compound silymarin, which has potent antioxidant and liver-protective

effects. Silymarin supports liver function, enhances detoxification, and promotes cellular regeneration.

3. **Turmeric**: Curcumin, the active compound in turmeric, exhibits anti-inflammatory, antioxidant, and liver-supportive properties. Turmeric aids in detoxification by enhancing liver function, reducing inflammation, and scavenging free radicals.

4. **Ginger**: Ginger is known for its digestive and anti-inflammatory properties, making it a valuable addition to herbal juices for detoxification. Ginger stimulates digestion, relieves nausea, and supports liver and gallbladder function.

5. **Leafy Greens**: Leafy greens such as kale, spinach, and Swiss chard are rich in chlorophyll, vitamins, minerals, and antioxidants that support detoxification and renewal. Chlorophyll helps cleanse the blood, alkalize the body, and promote cellular repair and regeneration.

Sample Herbal Juicing Recipes for Detoxification

1. **Liver Detox Green Juice**

   - Ingredients: Kale, spinach, cucumber, celery, lemon, ginger, dandelion greens

   - Instructions: Juice all ingredients together and enjoy immediately.

2. Golden Turmeric Detox Elixir

- Ingredients: Carrot, apple, turmeric root, ginger root, lemon, black pepper

- Instructions: Juice carrots, apples, turmeric, and ginger together. Squeeze lemon juice and add a pinch of black pepper. Stir well and enjoy.

3. Green Goddess Detox Smoothie

- Ingredients: Spinach, avocado, pineapple, cucumber, mint, coconut water

- Instructions: Blend all ingredients until smooth and creamy. Add coconut water to reach desired consistency. Pour into a glass and enjoy.

4. Liver-Cleansing Beet Juice

- Ingredients: Beets, carrots, apple, lemon, ginger, parsley

- Instructions: Juice beets, carrots, apple, lemon, ginger, and parsley together. Stir well and enjoy immediately.

5. Refreshing Cucumber Mint Detox Water

- Ingredients: Cucumber slices, mint leaves, lemon slices, filtered water

- Instructions: Combine cucumber slices, mint leaves, and lemon slices in a pitcher of filtered water. Allow to infuse for a few hours or overnight. Serve chilled and enjoy throughout the day.

Conclusion

Herbal juicing is a powerful tool for supporting the body's detoxification and renewal processes, providing essential nutrients, antioxidants, and liver-supportive compounds that promote cellular cleansing and regeneration. By incorporating key ingredients such as dandelion root, milk thistle, turmeric, ginger, and leafy greens into your juicing routine, you can enhance detoxification, support liver health, and rejuvenate your body from the inside out. Experiment with different herbal juice recipes to find combinations that resonate with your taste preferences and health goals, and embrace the transformative benefits of herbal juicing for detoxification and renewal.

CHAPTER SEVEN

Boosting Immunity Naturally: Herbs and Nutrients That Strengthen the Body's Defenses

A robust immune system is essential for protecting the body against infections, viruses, and other pathogens. While there is no magic bullet for boosting immunity, incorporating certain herbs and nutrients into your diet can help strengthen the body's natural defenses and support overall immune function. In this guide, we'll explore a variety of herbs and nutrients known for their immune-boosting properties, along with practical ways to incorporate them into your daily routine.

1. Echinacea

Echinacea is a popular herb known for its immune-stimulating properties. It contains active compounds such as polysaccharides and alkylamides that enhance the activity of immune cells and promote the production of cytokines, proteins involved in the immune response. Echinacea can be consumed as a tea, tincture, or supplement to support immune function during times of stress or illness.

2. Elderberry

Elderberry is rich in antioxidants and flavonoids, which have been shown to boost immune function and reduce the severity and duration of colds and flu. Elderberry extract is commonly used as a natural remedy for respiratory infections and can be taken in syrup or capsule form. It's important to note that elderberry supplements should be taken with caution, especially in high doses or for prolonged periods.

3. Astragalus

Astragalus is a traditional Chinese herb known for its immune-enhancing properties. It contains polysaccharides and saponins that stimulate the production of white blood cells and enhance the body's resistance to infections. Astragalus can be consumed as a tea, tincture, or supplement to support immune function and promote overall vitality.

4. Garlic

Garlic is prized for its immune-boosting and antimicrobial properties. It contains sulfur compounds such as allicin, which have been shown to enhance immune function, reduce inflammation, and inhibit the growth of harmful bacteria and viruses. Incorporating fresh garlic into your diet regularly can help support immune health and protect against infections.

5. Vitamin C

Vitamin C is a powerful antioxidant that plays a crucial role in immune function. It helps stimulate the production of white blood cells, which are essential for fighting off infections. Consuming foods rich in vitamin C, such as citrus fruits, bell peppers, kiwi, and broccoli, can help support immune function and reduce the risk of infections.

6. Vitamin D

Vitamin D is known as the "sunshine vitamin" because it is produced by the skin in response to sunlight exposure. It plays a critical role in immune function by modulating the activity of immune cells and reducing inflammation. Many people are deficient in vitamin D, especially during the winter months, so supplementation may be necessary to support immune health.

7. Zinc

Zinc is an essential mineral that plays a key role in immune function and wound healing. It helps regulate the activity of immune cells and supports the production of antibodies, which are essential for fighting off infections. Foods rich in zinc include oysters, beef, poultry, beans, and nuts.

Practical Tips for Boosting Immunity Naturally

1. **Eat a Balanced Diet**: Focus on whole, nutrient-dense foods such as fruits, vegetables, whole grains, lean proteins, and healthy fats to provide your body with essential vitamins, minerals, and antioxidants.

2. **Stay Hydrated**: Drink plenty of water throughout the day to keep your body hydrated and support optimal immune

function. Herbal teas, such as echinacea or ginger tea, can also provide hydration and immune-boosting benefits.

3. **Get Adequate Sleep**: Prioritize quality sleep to allow your body to rest, repair, and recharge. Aim for 7-9 hours of sleep per night to support immune health and overall well-being.

4. **Manage Stress**: Chronic stress can weaken the immune system and make you more susceptible to infections. Practice stress-reducing techniques such as meditation, deep breathing, yoga, or spending time in nature to promote relaxation and immune resilience.

5. **Stay Active**: Regular exercise can help boost immune function, reduce inflammation, and promote overall health. Aim for at least 30 minutes of moderate-intensity exercise most days of the week.

6. **Practice Good Hygiene**: Wash your hands frequently with soap and water, especially before eating or touching your face. Avoid close contact with sick individuals and practice respiratory hygiene by covering your mouth and nose when coughing or sneezing.

By incorporating these immune-boosting herbs and nutrients into your daily routine and adopting healthy lifestyle habits, you can strengthen your body's defenses and support optimal immune function. Remember that maintaining a strong immune system is a lifelong journey, so focus on making sustainable changes that promote overall health and well-being.

CHAPTER EIGHT

Overcoming Challenges: Tips for Successfully Completing the 7-Day Herbal Juicing Program

Embarking on a 7-day herbal juicing program can be a rewarding experience for your health and well-being, but it may also present challenges along the way. From managing cravings to navigating social situations, staying committed to your juicing journey requires determination, resilience, and a proactive approach. In this guide, we'll explore practical tips and strategies for overcoming common challenges and successfully completing the 7-day herbal juicing program.

1. Set Clear Goals and Intentions

Before starting the juicing program, take some time to reflect on your goals and intentions. What do you hope to achieve by completing the 7-day program? Whether it's detoxification, weight loss, or simply improving your overall health, setting clear goals will help you stay focused and motivated throughout the week.

2. Plan Ahead

Preparation is key to success when undertaking a juicing program. Take time to plan your juicing recipes, create a shopping list, and stock up on fresh fruits, vegetables, and herbs. Consider prepping your ingredients in advance to streamline the juicing process and ensure you have everything you need for the week ahead.

3. Stay Hydrated

Proper hydration is essential during the juicing program to support detoxification and overall well-being. In addition to drinking your herbal juices, be sure to drink plenty of water throughout the day to stay hydrated. Herbal teas and coconut water are also excellent hydrating options.

4. Manage Cravings

It's natural to experience cravings, especially in the early stages of the juicing program. To manage cravings, try incorporating small amounts of healthy fats and proteins into your diet, such as avocado, nuts, seeds, or plant-based protein powders. These can help stabilize blood sugar levels and keep you feeling satisfied between juices.

5. Listen to Your Body

Pay attention to how your body responds to the juicing program and adjust accordingly. If you're feeling fatigued or lightheaded, it may be a sign that you need to consume more calories or fluids. Similarly, if you're experiencing digestive discomfort, consider adding more fiber-rich ingredients to your juices or incorporating herbal teas to support digestion.

6. Stay Mindful and Present

Practicing mindfulness can help you stay present and focused during the juicing program, especially when faced with challenges or temptations. Take time to savor each sip of your herbal juices, appreciate the nourishment they provide, and cultivate gratitude for the opportunity to support your health and well-being.

7. Seek Support

Don't hesitate to reach out for support from friends, family, or online communities who can offer encouragement, accountability, and advice. Having a support system can make a significant difference in your ability to successfully complete the juicing program and overcome any obstacles that may arise.

8. Be Flexible and Adapt

Flexibility is key when navigating the ups and downs of a 7-day juicing program. If you encounter challenges or setbacks, don't be too hard on yourself. Instead, focus on finding creative solutions, adapting your approach as needed, and staying committed to your health goals.

9. Celebrate Your Achievements

Take time to celebrate your achievements and milestones throughout the juicing program. Whether it's completing a full day of juicing, trying a new recipe, or noticing improvements in your energy levels and well-being, every small victory deserves recognition and celebration.

10. Transition Mindfully

As you approach the end of the 7-day juicing program, transition back to solid foods mindfully and gradually. Start by incorporating light, easy-to-digest foods such as fruits, vegetables, and soups, and pay attention to how your body responds. Use this opportunity to reflect on what you've learned during the juicing program and how you can continue to prioritize your health and well-being moving forward.

By following these practical tips and strategies, you can overcome challenges and successfully complete the 7-day herbal juicing program with confidence and resilience. Remember that the journey to better health is not always easy, but with determination, support, and a positive mindset, you can achieve your goals and experience the transformative benefits of herbal juicing.

CHAPTER NINE

Inspiring Stories of Transformation: Real-Life Experiences of Cancer Remission Through Dr. Barbara's Protocol

Dr. Barbara's Herbal Juicing Protocol for Cancer Healing has garnered attention and acclaim for its holistic approach to supporting cancer patients on their healing journeys. While individual experiences may vary, there have been numerous inspiring stories of individuals who have achieved remarkable results and even remission from cancer through the implementation of Dr. Barbara's protocol. Here are a few real-life accounts of individuals who have experienced transformation and hope through Dr. Barbara's protocol:

1. Sarah's Journey to Remission

Sarah was diagnosed with stage 3 breast cancer and faced daunting treatment options, including chemotherapy, radiation, and surgery. Determined to explore alternative approaches, Sarah discovered Dr. Barbara's Herbal Juicing Protocol through a friend's recommendation. With the guidance of a holistic healthcare practitioner, Sarah began incorporating Dr. Barbara's cancer-fighting juices into her daily routine alongside other complementary therapies.

Over time, Sarah noticed significant improvements in her energy levels, mood, and overall well-being. Her oncologist was astounded by her progress during follow-up appointments, noting positive changes in her bloodwork and tumor markers. After several months of dedicated juicing and lifestyle changes, Sarah received the incredible news that her tumors had shrunk, and she was in remission. Today, Sarah continues to prioritize her health with regular juicing, mindful eating, and holistic self-care practices.

2. David's Triumph Over Prostate Cancer

David's journey with prostate cancer led him on a quest for natural healing modalities that complemented conventional treatments. Upon discovering Dr. Barbara's Herbal Juicing Protocol, David was intrigued by its focus on nourishing the body with nutrient-dense juices and herbal remedies. With the support of his healthcare team, David embarked on a personalized juicing regimen tailored to his specific health needs.

Through consistent juicing, dietary modifications, and stress-reduction techniques, David experienced profound shifts in his health and vitality. His energy levels soared, and he noticed a significant reduction in cancer-related symptoms such as fatigue and pain. Encouraged by his progress, David underwent regular medical evaluations, which revealed a remarkable improvement in his prostate health and overall well-being. Today, David attributes much of his success to Dr. Barbara's protocol and continues to share his story to inspire others on their healing journeys.

3. Lisa's Healing Journey with Leukemia

Lisa's battle with leukemia left her feeling overwhelmed and uncertain about her future. Determined to take an active role in her healing process, Lisa explored integrative approaches to cancer care and discovered Dr. Barbara's Herbal Juicing Protocol. Intrigued by the potential of herbal juices to support immune function and detoxification, Lisa began incorporating Dr. Barbara's recipes into her daily routine.

As she embraced a holistic lifestyle centered around juicing, nutrient-rich foods, and stress management techniques, Lisa noticed gradual improvements in her health and vitality. Her energy levels increased, and she experienced fewer side effects from her leukemia treatments. Over time, Lisa's medical scans showed a reduction in cancerous cells and markers, indicating a positive response to the juicing protocol.

Encouraged by her progress, Lisa became an advocate for holistic cancer care and shared her story with others facing similar challenges. Today, Lisa continues to prioritize her health and well-being with regular juicing, mindful living, and a deep sense of gratitude for the transformative power of Dr. Barbara's protocol.

Conclusion

These inspiring stories of transformation offer hope and encouragement to cancer patients seeking alternative approaches to healing. While Dr. Barbara's Herbal Juicing Protocol is not a cure-all, it has provided a supportive framework for many individuals on their journey to remission and improved quality of life. By combining the power of nutrient-dense juices with holistic lifestyle practices, individuals like Sarah, David, and Lisa have demonstrated the potential for profound healing and transformation in the face of cancer. As their stories illustrate, with dedication, perseverance, and the right support, anything is possible on the path to wellness and vitality.

CHAPTER TEN

Embracing a Healthier Lifestyle: Integrating Herbal Juicing into Your Ongoing Wellness Routine for Cancer Prevention and Long-Term Health

Incorporating herbal juicing into your ongoing wellness routine can be a powerful strategy for cancer prevention and long-term health. By nourishing your body with nutrient-rich juices and supporting its natural detoxification processes, you can strengthen your immune system, reduce inflammation, and promote overall vitality. In this guide, we'll explore practical tips and strategies for integrating herbal juicing into your daily life to support cancer prevention and long-term well-being.

1. Make Herbal Juicing a Daily Habit

Consistency is key when it comes to reaping the benefits of herbal juicing. Make it a daily habit to incorporate fresh, organic juices into your morning routine or as a midday pick-me-up. Set aside time each day to prepare and enjoy your juices, and consider investing in a high-quality juicer to make the process quick and convenient.

2. Experiment with a Variety of Ingredients

Keep your herbal juicing routine exciting and diverse by experimenting with a wide range of fruits, vegetables, and herbs. Incorporate seasonal produce and explore different flavor combinations to keep your taste buds engaged. Don't be afraid to get creative and try new ingredients, such as leafy greens, citrus fruits, ginger, turmeric, and herbs like parsley, cilantro, and mint.

3. Prioritize Nutrient-Dense Ingredients

Focus on incorporating nutrient-dense ingredients into your herbal juices to maximize their health benefits. Choose fruits and vegetables that are rich in vitamins, minerals, antioxidants, and phytonutrients, such as leafy greens, berries, citrus fruits, carrots, beets, and cruciferous vegetables. Consider adding superfoods like spirulina, chlorella, wheatgrass, and hemp seeds for an extra nutritional boost.

4. Tailor Your Juices to Your Health Needs

Customize your herbal juicing recipes to address specific health concerns or goals. For cancer prevention, focus on incorporating ingredients with anti-inflammatory, antioxidant, and immune-boosting properties, such as turmeric, ginger, garlic, green tea, and cruciferous vegetables. Consult with a holistic healthcare practitioner to develop personalized juicing recipes tailored to your individual health needs and preferences.

5. Practice Mindful Eating and Drinking

Approach herbal juicing with mindfulness and intention, paying attention to the flavors, textures, and sensations of each sip. Take time to savor and appreciate the nourishment your juices provide, and avoid rushing through meals or drinking mindlessly. Eating and drinking mindfully can enhance digestion, absorption, and enjoyment of your herbal juices, leading to greater satisfaction and satiety.

6. Support Your Juicing Routine with a Healthy Lifestyle

Incorporate herbal juicing into a holistic approach to health and wellness by adopting other healthy lifestyle habits. Prioritize regular physical activity, adequate sleep, stress management techniques, and mindful eating practices to support your overall well-being. By addressing multiple aspects of health, you can create a strong foundation for cancer prevention and long-term vitality.

7. Stay Informed and Inspired

Stay informed about the latest research and developments in herbal medicine, nutrition, and cancer prevention to continually refine and enhance your juicing routine. Seek out reputable sources of information, attend workshops or seminars, and connect with like-minded individuals who share your passion for natural health and healing. Surround yourself with positive influences and inspiring stories to stay motivated on your wellness journey.

Conclusion

Integrating herbal juicing into your ongoing wellness routine is a proactive and empowering step toward cancer prevention and long-term health. By nourishing your body with nutrient-rich juices, supporting its natural detoxification processes, and adopting a holistic approach to wellness, you can strengthen your immune system, reduce inflammation, and promote overall vitality. Embrace herbal juicing as a delicious and convenient way to prioritize your health and well-being, and let it serve as a cornerstone of your journey toward optimal health and longevity.

CHAPTER 11
JUICING RECIPES FOR CANCER

1. Turmeric Juice:

- **Definition:** Turmeric contains curcumin, known for its anti-inflammatory and antioxidant properties, which may help in fighting cancer.

- **Ingredients:** Fresh turmeric root, ginger, lemon, honey, water.

- **Preparation:** Blend turmeric root, ginger, lemon juice, honey, and water until smooth.

- **How to Use:** Drink a small glass daily.

- **Dosage:** 1 glass per day.

- **Side Effects:** May cause gastrointestinal issues in some individuals.

- **Precautions:** Avoid excessive consumption, especially if on blood-thinning medications.

2. Aloe Vera Juice:

- **Definition:** Aloe vera contains compounds with potential anti-cancer properties and helps in detoxification.

- **Ingredients:** Aloe vera gel, lemon juice, honey, water.

- Preparation: Blend aloe vera gel, lemon juice, honey, and water until well combined.

- How to Use: Consume a small glass daily, preferably in the morning.

- Dosage: 1 glass per day.

- Side Effects: May cause digestive discomfort in some individuals.

- Precautions: Consult a healthcare professional if pregnant or breastfeeding.

3. Wheatgrass Juice:

- Definition: Wheatgrass is rich in chlorophyll and antioxidants, which may help in detoxification and fighting cancer.

- Ingredients: Fresh wheatgrass, water.

- Preparation: Juice fresh wheatgrass using a juicer.

- How to Use: Drink immediately after juicing.

- Dosage: 1-2 ounces per day.

- Side Effects: May cause nausea or allergic reactions in some individuals.

- Precautions: Start with a small amount to check for any adverse reactions.

4. Ginger Juice:

- **Definition:** Ginger contains gingerol, which exhibits anti-inflammatory and antioxidant properties, potentially aiding in cancer prevention.

- **Ingredients:** Fresh ginger, lemon juice, honey, water.

- **Preparation:** Blend fresh ginger, lemon juice, honey, and water until smooth.

- **How to Use:** Consume a small glass daily, preferably before meals.

- **Dosage:** 1 glass per day.

- **Side Effects:** May cause heartburn or digestive issues in some individuals.

- **Precautions:** Avoid excessive consumption, especially if prone to gallstones.

5. Garlic Juice:

- **Definition:** Garlic contains allicin, which exhibits anti-cancer properties and boosts the immune system.

- **Ingredients:** Fresh garlic cloves, lemon juice, honey, water.

- **Preparation:** Blend garlic cloves, lemon juice, honey, and water until well combined.

- How to Use: Consume a small glass daily.

- Dosage: 1 glass per day.

- Side Effects: May cause bad breath or digestive discomfort.

- Precautions: Consult a healthcare professional if on blood-thinning medications.

6. Green Tea Juice:

- Definition: Green tea contains catechins, which have antioxidant properties and may help in cancer prevention.

- Ingredients: Green tea leaves, lemon juice, honey, water.

- Preparation: Brew green tea and let it cool, then blend with lemon juice, honey, and water.

- How to Use: Drink a small glass daily.

- Dosage: 1 glass per day.

- Side Effects: May cause insomnia or jitteriness due to caffeine content.

- Precautions: Avoid consuming excessive amounts, especially if sensitive to caffeine.

7. Beetroot Juice:

- Definition: Beetroot contains betalains, which have antioxidant properties and may help in detoxification and cancer prevention.

- Ingredients: Fresh beetroot, carrot, apple, lemon juice.

- Preparation: Juice beetroot, carrot, apple, and lemon juice together.

- How to Use: Drink immediately after juicing.

- Dosage: 1 glass per day.

- Side Effects: May cause red urine or stool.

- Precautions: Start with a small amount to avoid digestive discomfort.

8. Carrot Juice:

- Definition: Carrots are rich in beta-carotene, which converts to vitamin A in the body and exhibits antioxidant properties.

- Ingredients: Fresh carrots, ginger, lemon juice, honey, water.

- Preparation: Juice carrots, ginger, lemon juice, honey, and water together.

- How to Use: Consume a small glass daily.

- Dosage: 1 glass per day.

- Side Effects: May cause yellowing of the skin (carotenemia) if consumed excessively.

- Precautions: Monitor for allergic reactions, especially if allergic to carrots.

9. Parsley Juice:

- Definition: Parsley contains flavonoids and volatile oils, which have antioxidant and anti-inflammatory properties.

- Ingredients: Fresh parsley, cucumber, lemon juice, honey, water.

- Preparation: Blend parsley, cucumber, lemon juice, honey, and water until smooth.

- How to Use: Drink a small glass daily.

- Dosage: 1 glass per day.

- Side Effects: May cause allergic reactions in some individuals.

- Precautions: Avoid excessive consumption, especially if prone to kidney stones.

10. Holy Basil (Tulsi) Juice:

- Definition: Holy basil contains eugenol, which exhibits anti-inflammatory and antioxidant properties and may help in cancer prevention.

- Ingredients: Fresh holy basil leaves, lemon juice, honey, water.

- Preparation: Blend holy basil leaves, lemon juice, honey, and water until well combined.

- How to Use: Consume a small glass daily.

- Dosage: 1 glass per day.

- Side Effects: May cause hypoglycemia in some individuals.

- Precautions: Monitor blood sugar levels, especially if diabetic.

11. Lemon Juice:

- Definition: Lemon juice is rich in vitamin C and antioxidants, which may help in boosting the immune system and fighting cancer.

- Ingredients: Fresh lemon juice, honey, water.

- Preparation: Mix fresh lemon juice with honey and water.

- How to Use: Drink a small glass daily, preferably in the morning.

- Dosage: 1 glass per day.

- Side Effects: May cause tooth enamel erosion if consumed excessively.

- Precautions: Rinse mouth with water after consumption to protect teeth.

12. **Moringa Juice:**

- Definition: Moringa leaves are rich in antioxidants, vitamins, and minerals, which may help in boosting the immune system and fighting cancer.

- Ingredients: Fresh moringa leaves, lemon juice, honey, water.

- Preparation: Blend moringa leaves, lemon juice, honey, and water until smooth.

- How to Use: Consume a small glass daily.

- Dosage: 1 glass per day.

- Side Effects: May cause digestive discomfort in some individuals.

- Precautions: Avoid excessive consumption, especially if prone to hypoglycemia.

13. **Cranberry Juice:**

- **Definition:** Cranberries contain proanthocyanidins, which have antioxidant properties and may help in preventing certain types of cancer.

- **Ingredients:** Fresh cranberries, apple, lemon juice, honey, water.

- **Preparation:** Blend cranberries, apple, lemon juice, honey, and water until well combined.

- **How to Use:** Consume a small glass daily.

- **Dosage:** 1 glass per day.

- **Side Effects:** May cause gastrointestinal upset in some individuals.

- **Precautions:** Avoid if prone to kidney stones due to oxalate content.

14. **Soursop (Graviola) Juice:**

- **Definition:** Soursop contains acetogenins, which have been studied for their potential anti-cancer properties.

- **Ingredients:** Fresh soursop pulp, pineapple, lime juice, honey, water.

- **Preparation:** Blend soursop pulp, pineapple, lime juice, honey, and water until smooth.

- How to Use: Consume a small glass daily.

- Dosage: 1 glass per day.

- Side Effects: May cause nausea or allergic reactions in some individuals.

- Precautions: Avoid excessive consumption, especially if prone to hypoglycemia.

15. Grape Juice:

- Definition: Grapes contain resveratrol, which exhibits antioxidant properties and may help in cancer prevention.

- Ingredients: Fresh grapes, lemon juice, honey, water.

- Preparation: Blend grapes, lemon juice, honey, and water until well combined.

- How to Use: Consume a small glass daily.

- Dosage: 1 glass per day.

- Side Effects: May cause digestive discomfort in some individuals.

- Precautions: Monitor blood sugar levels, especially if diabetic.

SOME HERBAL REMEDIES YOU SHOULD KNOW

Blue Vervain:

Definition: Blue vervain, also known as Verbena hastata, is a perennial herb native to North America. It has been used in traditional medicine for centuries to treat various ailments, including anxiety, insomnia, and digestive issues.

Ingredients: Blue vervain contains several active compounds, including aucubin, verbenalin, and volatile oils. These compounds are believed to contribute to the herb's medicinal properties.

How to Prepare: Blue vervain is typically consumed as a tea or tincture. To make tea, dried blue vervain leaves and flowers are steeped in hot water for several minutes before being strained and consumed. Tinctures are prepared by steeping the herb in alcohol or vinegar to extract its active compounds.

Dosage: The appropriate dosage of blue vervain can vary depending on factors such as age, health status, and the specific preparation being used. It's important to follow the recommended dosage on the product label or consult with a qualified herbalist or healthcare professional for personalized guidance.

How to Use: Blue vervain tea or tincture is typically taken orally. It can be consumed on its own or mixed with honey or other herbal teas for added flavor.

Side Effects: While blue vervain is generally considered safe for most people when used in moderation, excessive intake may cause digestive upset or allergic reactions in some individuals. Pregnant or breastfeeding women should avoid blue vervain due to its potential to stimulate uterine contractions. As with any herbal remedy, it's important to consult with a healthcare provider before using blue vervain, especially if you have underlying health conditions or are taking medications.

Bromide Plus Powder:

Definition: Bromide Plus Powder is a dietary supplement formulated to support thyroid health and promote overall well-being. It typically contains a blend of herbs and minerals that are believed to have beneficial effects on thyroid function.

Ingredients: Bromide Plus Powder often contains a combination of herbs such as bladderwrack, sea moss, and burdock root, along with minerals like iodine and potassium phosphate. These ingredients are thought to support thyroid function and maintain optimal iodine levels in the body.

How to Prepare: Bromide Plus Powder is usually mixed with water or juice to create a drinkable solution. It's important to follow the instructions on the product label for dosage and preparation.

Dosage: The dosage of Bromide Plus Powder can vary depending on the specific product and individual needs. It's crucial to consult with a healthcare professional or follow the recommended dosage on the product label to avoid potential side effects.

How to Use: Bromide Plus Powder is typically taken orally by mixing the recommended dosage with water or juice. It's important to shake or stir the mixture well before consuming it to ensure even distribution of the ingredients.

Side Effects: While Bromide Plus Powder is generally considered safe when used as directed, some individuals may experience side effects such as digestive discomfort or allergic reactions to certain ingredients. It's essential to consult with a healthcare provider before starting any new supplement regimen, especially if you have underlying health conditions or are taking medications.

Bugleweed:

Definition: Bugleweed, also known as Lycopusvirginicus, is a perennial herb native to North America and Europe. It has been used in traditional medicine to treat various conditions, including hyperthyroidism, anxiety, and insomnia.

Ingredients: Bugleweed contains several active compounds, including lithospermic acid, phenolic acids, and flavonoids. These compounds are believed to contribute to the herb's medicinal properties, particularly its ability to regulate thyroid function.

How to Prepare: Bugleweed is commonly consumed as a tea or tincture. To make tea, dried bugleweed leaves and flowers are steeped in hot water for several minutes before being strained and consumed. Tinctures are prepared by steeping the herb in alcohol or vinegar to extract its active compounds.

Dosage: The appropriate dosage of bugleweed can vary depending on factors such as age, health status, and the specific preparation being used. It's important to follow the recommended dosage on the product label or consult with a qualified herbalist or healthcare professional for personalized guidance.

How to Use: Bugleweed tea or tincture is typically taken orally. It can be consumed on its own or mixed with honey or other herbal teas for added flavor.

Side Effects: While bugleweed is generally considered safe for most people when used in moderation, excessive intake may cause digestive upset or allergic reactions in some individuals. Pregnant or breastfeeding women should avoid bugleweed due to its potential to stimulate uterine contractions. As with any herbal remedy, it's important to consult with a healthcare provider before using bugleweed, especially if you have underlying health conditions or are taking medications.

Burdock:

Definition: Burdock, scientifically known as Arctium lappa, is a biennial plant native to Europe and Asia but now found worldwide. It's part of the Asteraceae family and has been used for centuries in traditional medicine and culinary practices.

Ingredients: Burdock contains various nutrients, including carbohydrates, fiber, vitamins (such as vitamin B6, folate, and vitamin C), and minerals (including potassium, magnesium, and manganese). It also contains active compounds such as polyphenols and volatile oils.

How to Prepare: Burdock can be prepared and consumed in various ways. The roots, leaves, and seeds are all utilized for different purposes. The root is commonly used in cooking, herbal teas, tinctures, and supplements, while the leaves and seeds are sometimes used in herbal preparations.

Dosage: The appropriate dosage of burdock root can vary depending on the specific form and intended use. For culinary purposes, there are no strict dosage guidelines, but for supplements or herbal remedies, it's essential to follow the recommended dosage on the product label or consult with a healthcare professional.

How to Use: Burdock root can be used in cooking by peeling, slicing, and adding it to soups, stews, stir-fries, or salads. It can also be brewed into a tea or used to make tinctures or extracts for medicinal purposes. Some people may also take burdock root supplements in capsule or powder form.

Side Effects: While burdock is generally considered safe for most people when consumed in moderate amounts, some individuals may experience allergic reactions or digestive upset. Additionally, burdock may interact with certain medications or have adverse effects in individuals with certain health conditions, such as diabetes or allergies to plants in the Asteraceae family. It's important to consult with a healthcare provider before using burdock, especially if you have underlying health conditions or are taking medications.

Cascara Sagrada:

Definition: Cascara Sagrada, scientifically known as Rhamnus purshiana, is a species of buckthorn native to western North America. It has been used traditionally as a laxative and to promote bowel regularity.

Ingredients: The primary active ingredients in cascara sagrada are anthraquinone glycosides, particularly cascarosides A and B. These compounds stimulate peristalsis in the colon, leading to increased bowel movements.

How to Prepare: Cascara sagrada is typically prepared as an herbal tea, tincture, or capsule. To make tea, dried cascara sagrada bark is steeped in hot water for several minutes before being strained and consumed. Tinctures are prepared by steeping the bark in alcohol to extract its active compounds.

Dosage: The appropriate dosage of cascara sagrada can vary depending on the specific preparation and intended use. It's important to follow the recommended dosage on the product label or consult with a healthcare professional for personalized guidance.

How to Use: Cascara sagrada tea or tincture is typically taken orally. It's important to start with a low dose and gradually increase if needed to avoid potential side effects such as cramping or diarrhea.

Side Effects: Cascara sagrada is considered safe for short-term use when used as directed. However, long-term or excessive use may lead to dependence, electrolyte imbalance, or dehydration. It may also interact with certain medications or have adverse effects in individuals with certain health conditions. It's important to use cascara sagrada under the guidance of a healthcare professional and to discontinue use if any adverse effects occur.

Cell Food:

Definition: Cell Food is a dietary supplement marketed as a highly oxygenating and alkalizing formula. It's claimed to support overall health and vitality by providing essential nutrients and oxygen to the cells.

Ingredients: The exact ingredients of Cell Food can vary depending on the brand, but it typically contains a proprietary blend of minerals, enzymes, electrolytes, and trace elements. Some common ingredients may include purified water, dissolved oxygen, seawater extract, and plant-based enzymes.

How to Prepare: Cell Food is usually available in liquid form and is typically taken orally. It can be consumed directly or diluted in water or juice before consumption.

Dosage: The dosage of Cell Food can vary depending on the specific product and individual needs. It's important to follow the recommended dosage on the product label or consult with a healthcare professional for personalized guidance.

How to Use: Cell Food is typically taken orally, either directly or mixed into water or juice. It's important to shake the bottle well before use and to store it according to the manufacturer's instructions.

Side Effects: Cell Food is generally considered safe for most people when used as directed. However, some individuals may experience mild digestive upset or allergic reactions to certain ingredients. It's essential to consult with a healthcare provider before starting any new supplement regimen, especially if you have underlying health conditions or are taking medications.

Chaparral:

Definition: Chaparral, scientifically known as Larrea tridentata, is a shrub native to the southwestern United States and northern Mexico. It has been used for centuries by Native American tribes for its medicinal properties and is commonly used in herbal medicine today.

Ingredients: Chaparral contains several bioactive compounds, including nordihydroguaiaretic acid (NDGA), flavonoids, lignans, and volatile oils. NDGA is believed to be the primary active compound responsible for many of chaparral's therapeutic effects.

How to Prepare: Chaparral can be prepared and consumed in various forms, including teas, tinctures, capsules, and topical preparations. To make tea, dried chaparral leaves are steeped in hot water for several minutes before being strained and consumed. Tinctures are prepared by steeping the herb in alcohol or vinegar to extract its active compounds.

Dosage: The appropriate dosage of chaparral can vary depending on the specific form and intended use. It's important to follow the recommended dosage on the product label or consult with a healthcare professional for personalized guidance.

How to Use: Chaparral tea or tincture is typically taken orally. It can also be applied topically to the skin for certain conditions. It's important to use chaparral products as directed and to discontinue use if any adverse effects occur.

Side Effects: Chaparral is generally considered safe for most people when used in moderate amounts. However, excessive intake or prolonged use may lead to liver toxicity or other adverse effects. It may also interact with certain medications or have adverse effects in individuals with certain health conditions. It's important to use chaparral under the guidance of a healthcare professional and to discontinue use if any adverse effects occur.

Cocolmeca:

Definition: Cocolmeca, also known as Smilax ornata or sarsaparilla, is a flowering vine native to Mexico and Central America. It has been used traditionally in Mexican and Central American folk medicine for its purported medicinal properties.

Ingredients: Cocolmeca contains various bioactive compounds, including saponins, flavonoids, and plant sterols. These compounds are believed to contribute to the herb's medicinal properties, including its potential as a diuretic, blood purifier, and anti-inflammatory agent.

How to Prepare: Cocolmeca is commonly prepared and consumed as an herbal tea or decoction. To make tea, dried cocolmeca roots or leaves are steeped in hot water for several minutes before being strained and consumed. Decoctions involve boiling the roots or leaves in water to extract their active compounds.

Dosage: The appropriate dosage of cocolmeca can vary depending on factors such as age, health status, and the specific preparation being used. It's important to follow the recommended dosage on the product label or consult with a qualified herbalist or healthcare professional for personalized guidance.

How to Use: Cocolmeca tea or decoction is typically taken orally. It can also be used topically for certain skin conditions. It's important to use cocolmeca products as directed and to discontinue use if any adverse effects occur.

Side Effects: Cocolmeca is generally considered safe for most people when used in moderate amounts. However, excessive intake may lead to digestive upset or other adverse effects. It may also interact with certain medications or have adverse effects in individuals with certain health conditions. It's important to use cocolmeca under the guidance of a healthcare professional and to discontinue use if any adverse effects occur.

Contribo:

Definition: Contribo, also known as Aristolochiatrilobata, is a vine native to the Caribbean and Central America. It has been used traditionally in folk medicine for various purposes, including as a remedy for digestive issues, inflammation, and pain relief.

Ingredients: Contribo contains several bioactive compounds, including aristolochic acids, flavonoids, and alkaloids. These compounds are believed to contribute to the herb's medicinal properties, including its potential as an anti-inflammatory and analgesic agent.

How to Prepare: Contribo is typically prepared and consumed as an herbal tea or decoction. To make tea, dried contribo leaves or stems are steeped in hot water for several minutes before being strained and consumed. Decoctions involve boiling the leaves or stems in water to extract their active compounds.

Dosage: The appropriate dosage of contribo can vary depending on factors such as age, health status, and the specific preparation being used. It's important to follow the recommended dosage on the product label or consult with a qualified herbalist or healthcare professional for personalized guidance.

How to Use: Contribo tea or decoction is typically taken orally. It's important to use contribo products as directed and to discontinue use if any adverse effects occur.

Side Effects: Contribo contains aristolochic acids, which have been associated with serious adverse effects, including kidney damage and cancer. Due to these safety concerns, the use of contribo is highly discouraged, and it's important to avoid products containing aristolochic acids. Individuals should seek alternative remedies for their health needs.

Dandelion Root:

Definition: Dandelion, scientifically known as Taraxacum officinale, is a common flowering plant found worldwide. While often considered a pesky weed, dandelion has a long history of use in traditional medicine for its various health benefits.

Ingredients: Dandelion root contains several bioactive compounds, including sesquiterpene lactones, triterpenes, flavonoids, and polysaccharides. These compounds are believed to contribute to the herb's medicinal properties, including its potential as a diuretic, digestive aid, and liver tonic.

How to Prepare: Dandelion root can be prepared and consumed in various forms, including teas, tinctures, capsules, and extracts. To make tea, dried dandelion root is steeped in hot water for several minutes before being strained and consumed. Tinctures are prepared by steeping the root in alcohol or vinegar to extract its active compounds.

Dosage: The appropriate dosage of dandelion root can vary depending on factors such as age, health status, and the specific preparation being used. It's important to follow the recommended dosage on the product label or consult with a qualified herbalist or healthcare professional for personalized guidance.

How to Use: Dandelion root tea, tincture, or capsules are typically taken orally. It's important to use dandelion root products as directed and to discontinue use if any adverse effects occur.

Side Effects: Dandelion root is generally considered safe for most people when used in moderate amounts. However, some individuals may experience allergic reactions or digestive upset. It may also interact with certain medications or have adverse effects in individuals with certain health conditions. It's important to use dandelion root under the guidance of a healthcare professional and to discontinue use if any adverse effects occur.

Green Food Plus:

Definition: Green Food Plus is a dietary supplement formulated to provide a concentrated source of nutrients derived from various green plants. It's designed to support overall health and well-being by delivering essential vitamins, minerals, antioxidants, and phytonutrients.

Ingredients: Green Food Plus typically contains a blend of powdered green vegetables, grasses, algae, and other plant-based ingredients. Common ingredients may include wheatgrass, barley grass, spirulina, chlorella, alfalfa, kale, spinach, and broccoli, among others.

How to Prepare: Green Food Plus is usually available in powder form and can be mixed with water, juice, or smoothies. It's important to follow the recommended dosage on the product label and to consume it as part of a balanced diet.

Dosage: The appropriate dosage of Green Food Plus can vary depending on the specific product and individual needs. It's important to follow the recommended dosage on the product label or consult with a healthcare professional for personalized guidance.

How to Use: Green Food Plus powder is typically mixed with water, juice, or smoothies and consumed orally. It's often taken once or twice daily, preferably with meals, to maximize nutrient absorption.

Side Effects: Green Food Plus is generally considered safe for most people when used as directed. However, some individuals may experience digestive upset or allergic reactions to certain ingredients. It's important to consult with a healthcare provider before starting any new supplement regimen, especially if you have underlying health conditions or are taking medications.

Guaco:

Definition: Guaco, also known as Mikania cordata or Mikania glomerata, is a medicinal plant native to Central and South America. It has a long history of use in traditional medicine for its potential therapeutic properties.

Ingredients: Guaco contains several bioactive compounds, including coumarins, flavonoids, tannins, and saponins. These compounds are believed to contribute to the herb's medicinal properties, including its potential as an expectorant, anti-inflammatory, and antispasmodic agent.

How to Prepare: Guaco is typically prepared and consumed as an herbal tea or infusion. To make tea, dried guaco leaves are steeped in hot water for several minutes before being strained and consumed.

Dosage: The appropriate dosage of guaco can vary depending on factors such as age, health status, and the specific preparation being used. It's important to follow the recommended dosage on the product label or consult with a qualified herbalist or healthcare professional for personalized guidance.

How to Use: Guaco tea is typically taken orally. It can be consumed on its own or mixed with honey or other herbal teas for added flavor.

Side Effects: Guaco is generally considered safe for most people when used in moderate amounts. However, some individuals may experience allergic reactions or digestive upset. It may also interact with certain medications or have adverse effects in individuals with certain health conditions. It's important to use guaco under the guidance of a healthcare professional and to discontinue use if any adverse effects occur.

Hydrangea:

Definition: Hydrangea, scientifically known as Hydrangea arborescens, is a flowering shrub native to North America. It has been used traditionally in herbal medicine for its potential diuretic and anti-inflammatory properties.

Ingredients: Hydrangea contains several bioactive compounds, including saponins, flavonoids, and glycosides. These compounds are believed to contribute to the herb's medicinal properties, including its potential as a diuretic, kidney tonic, and anti-inflammatory agent.

How to Prepare: Hydrangea root is typically prepared and consumed as an herbal tea or tincture. To make tea, dried hydrangea root is steeped in hot water for several minutes before being strained and consumed. Tinctures are prepared by steeping the root in alcohol or vinegar to extract its active compounds.

Dosage: The appropriate dosage of hydrangea can vary depending on factors such as age, health status, and the specific preparation being used. It's important to follow the recommended dosage on the product label or consult with a qualified herbalist or healthcare professional for personalized guidance.

How to Use: Hydrangea tea or tincture is typically taken orally. It's important to use hydrangea products as directed and to discontinue use if any adverse effects occur.

Side Effects: Hydrangea is generally considered safe for most people when used in moderate amounts. However, some individuals may experience digestive upset or allergic reactions. It may also interact with certain medications or have adverse effects in individuals with certain health conditions. It's important to use hydrangea under the guidance of a healthcare professional and to discontinue use if any adverse effects occur.

Lymphalin:

Definition: Lymphalin is a herbal supplement formulated to support lymphatic system health. The lymphatic system plays a crucial role in immune function and waste removal in the body, and Lymphalin is designed to promote its proper function.

Ingredients: Lymphalin typically contains a blend of herbs and botanical extracts known for their traditional use in supporting lymphatic system health. Common ingredients may include cleavers, red clover, echinacea, burdock root, and calendula, among others.

How to Prepare: Lymphalin is usually available in capsule or liquid form. Capsules are taken orally with water, while liquid forms may be mixed with water or juice before consumption. It's important to follow the recommended dosage on the product label.

Dosage: The appropriate dosage of Lymphalin can vary depending on the specific product and individual needs. It's important to follow the recommended dosage on the product label or consult with a healthcare professional for personalized guidance.

How to Use: Lymphalin capsules are typically taken orally with water, while liquid forms may be mixed with water or juice before consumption. It's often recommended to take Lymphalin on an empty stomach for optimal absorption.

Side Effects: Lymphalin is generally considered safe for most people when used as directed. However, some individuals may experience mild side effects such as gastrointestinal discomfort or allergic reactions to certain ingredients. It's important to consult with a healthcare provider before starting any new supplement regimen, especially if you have underlying health conditions or are taking medications.

Manjakani:

Definition: Manjakani, also known as Quercus infectoria or oak gall, is a natural substance derived from the oak tree. It has been used for centuries in traditional medicine for its potential health benefits, particularly for women's health and vaginal tightening.

Ingredients: Manjakani contains various bioactive compounds, including tannins, flavonoids, and gallic acid. These compounds are believed to contribute to the herb's medicinal properties, including its potential as an astringent and antiseptic agent.

How to Prepare: Manjakani is typically available in powder, capsule, or liquid extract form. It can be taken orally or used topically depending on the intended use. For vaginal tightening, manjakani may be applied topically as a gel or inserted into the vagina in capsule form.

Dosage: The appropriate dosage of manjakani can vary depending on factors such as age, health status, and the specific preparation being used. It's important to follow the recommended dosage on the product label or consult with a qualified herbalist or healthcare professional for personalized guidance.

How to Use: Manjakani can be taken orally or used topically depending on the intended use. It's important to use manjakani products as directed and to discontinue use if any adverse effects occur.

Side Effects: Manjakani is generally considered safe for most people when used in moderate amounts. However, some individuals may experience allergic reactions or skin irritation when used topically. It's important to use manjakani under the guidance of a healthcare professional and to discontinue use if any adverse effects occur.

Red Clover:

Definition: Red clover, scientifically known as Trifolium pratense, is a flowering plant belonging to the legume family. It's native to Europe, Western Asia, and Northwest Africa but has been naturalized in many other regions. Red clover has been used in traditional medicine for various purposes, including its potential to support women's health and menopausal symptoms.

Ingredients: Red clover contains several bioactive compounds, including isoflavones (such as genistein and daidzein), flavonoids, and phytoestrogens. These compounds are believed to contribute to the herb's medicinal properties, including its potential as a hormone-balancing agent and its ability to support cardiovascular health.

How to Prepare: Red clover is typically prepared and consumed as an herbal tea or tincture. To make tea, dried red clover flowers are steeped in hot water for several minutes before being strained and consumed. Tinctures are prepared by steeping the flowers in alcohol or vinegar to extract their active compounds.

Dosage: The appropriate dosage of red clover can vary depending on factors such as age, health status, and the specific preparation being used. It's important to follow the recommended dosage on the product label or consult with a qualified herbalist or healthcare professional for personalized guidance.

How to Use: Red clover tea or tincture is typically taken orally. It's important to use red clover products as directed and to discontinue use if any adverse effects occur.

Side Effects: Red clover is generally considered safe for most people when used in moderate amounts. However, some individuals may experience allergic reactions or digestive upset. It may also interact with certain medications or have adverse effects in individuals with certain health conditions. It's important to use red clover under the guidance of a healthcare professional and to discontinue use if any adverse effects occur.

Irish Moss:

Definition: Irish Moss, scientifically known as Chondrus crispus, is a species of red algae or seaweed native to the Atlantic coastlines of Europe and North America. It has been used for centuries in traditional Irish and Scottish cuisine, as well as in herbal medicine.

Ingredients: Irish Moss is rich in various nutrients, including iodine, sulfur compounds, vitamins (such as vitamin A, vitamin K, and vitamin B12), minerals (including calcium, magnesium, potassium, and sodium), and polysaccharides (such as carrageenan). These nutrients are believed to contribute to the herb's potential health benefits.

How to Prepare: Irish Moss is typically prepared by soaking it in water to rehydrate and soften it before use. It can be added to soups, stews, smoothies, desserts, and other dishes as a thickening agent or nutritional supplement.

Dosage: The appropriate dosage of Irish Moss can vary depending on factors such as age, health status, and the specific preparation being used. It's important to follow recipes or guidelines for culinary use and to consult with a healthcare professional for guidance on using Irish Moss as a dietary supplement.

How to Use: Irish Moss can be used in culinary applications to add thickness and nutritional value to dishes. It can also be consumed as a dietary supplement in the form of capsules, powders, or extracts.

Side Effects: Irish Moss is generally considered safe for most people when consumed in moderate amounts as part of a balanced diet. However, some individuals may be allergic to seaweed or carrageenan, a compound found in Irish Moss that is used as a food additive. It's important to discontinue use if any adverse effects occur and to consult with a healthcare professional if you have any concerns.

Irish Sea Moss:

Definition: Irish Sea Moss is a term often used interchangeably with Irish Moss, referring to the same species of red algae,

Chondrus crispus. It's harvested from the rocky shores of the Atlantic coastlines of Europe and North America.

Ingredients: Irish Sea Moss shares the same nutritional profile as Irish Moss, containing iodine, vitamins, minerals, and polysaccharides. It's valued for its potential health benefits, including supporting thyroid function, boosting immune health, and promoting digestion.

How to Prepare: Irish Sea Moss is prepared in the same way as Irish Moss, by soaking it in water to rehydrate and soften it before use. It can be used in culinary applications or consumed as a dietary supplement.

Dosage: The dosage of Irish Sea Moss depends on the form and intended use. As a dietary supplement, it's important to follow the recommended dosage on the product label or consult with a healthcare professional for personalized guidance.

How to Use: Irish Sea Moss can be used in various culinary applications, including soups, smoothies, desserts, and sauces. It can also be consumed as a dietary supplement in the form of capsules, powders, or extracts.

Side Effects: Similar to Irish Moss, Irish Sea Moss is generally considered safe for most people when consumed in moderate amounts. However, individuals with seaweed allergies or sensitivities to carrageenan should exercise caution. It's important to discontinue use if any adverse effects occur and to consult with a healthcare professional if you have any concerns.

Herban Iron:

Definition: Herban Iron is a dietary supplement designed to provide an easily absorbable form of iron to support healthy iron levels in the body. It's particularly beneficial for individuals with iron deficiency or anemia.

Ingredients: Herban Iron typically contains iron in the form of ferrous bisglycinate, which is a highly bioavailable and gentle form of iron that is less likely to cause digestive upset or constipation compared to other forms of iron. It may also contain other ingredients such as vitamin C to enhance iron absorption.

How to Prepare: Herban Iron is usually available in capsule or liquid form. Capsules are taken orally with water, while liquid forms may be mixed with water or juice before consumption. It's important to follow the recommended dosage on the product label.

Dosage: The appropriate dosage of Herban Iron depends on factors such as age, gender, and the severity of iron deficiency. It's important to consult with a healthcare professional to determine the correct dosage for individual needs.

How to Use: Herban Iron capsules are typically taken orally with water, while liquid forms may be mixed with water or juice before consumption. It's important to take Herban Iron as directed and to avoid taking it with dairy products, antacids, or other substances that may interfere with iron absorption.

Side Effects: While Herban Iron is generally considered safe for most people when used as directed, some individuals may experience mild side effects such as gastrointestinal discomfort or constipation. It's important to consult with a healthcare professional before starting any new supplement regimen, especially if you have underlying health conditions or are taking medications.

Bio Ferro Tonic:

Definition: Bio Ferro Tonic is a dietary supplement primarily composed of herbs and minerals. It's often marketed as a natural way to support overall health, particularly by promoting blood health and circulation.

Ingredients: Typical ingredients in Bio Ferro Tonic may include a blend of herbs such as burdock root, yellow dock root, sarsaparilla root, and cascara sagrada bark, along with minerals like iron and potassium phosphate.

How to Prepare: Bio Ferro Tonic usually comes in liquid form and is typically taken orally. It's important to follow the instructions on the product label for dosage and administration.

Dosage: The dosage can vary depending on the specific product and individual needs. It's crucial to consult with a healthcare professional or follow the recommended dosage on the product label to avoid potential side effects.

How to Use: Bio Ferro Tonic is often taken by adding the recommended dosage to water or juice and consuming it orally. It's important to shake the bottle well before use and store it according to the manufacturer's instructions.

Side Effects: While Bio Ferro Tonic is generally considered safe when used as directed, some individuals may experience side effects such as digestive discomfort, allergic reactions, or interactions with medications. It's essential to consult with a healthcare provider before starting any new supplement regimen, especially if you have underlying health conditions or are taking medications.

Bladderwrack:

Definition: Bladderwrack is a type of seaweed or marine algae commonly used in traditional medicine and as a dietary supplement. It's known for its potential health benefits, particularly related to thyroid health and weight management.

Ingredients: Bladderwrack contains various nutrients, including iodine, vitamins, minerals, and antioxidants. The primary active components are iodine and fucoidan, a type of carbohydrate found in brown seaweeds.

How to Prepare: Bladderwrack supplements are available in various forms, including capsules, powders, and liquid extracts. They can be taken orally with water or added to smoothies and other beverages.

Dosage: The appropriate dosage of bladderwrack can vary based on factors such as age, health status, and the specific product being used. It's essential to follow the recommended dosage on the product label or consult with a healthcare professional for personalized guidance.

How to Use: Bladderwrack supplements are typically taken orally, either with water or mixed into food or beverages. It's important to follow the instructions on the product label and avoid exceeding the recommended dosage.

Side Effects: While bladderwrack is generally considered safe for most people when used in moderation, excessive intake of iodine from bladderwrack supplements can cause thyroid dysfunction and other adverse effects. Individuals with thyroid disorders, iodine sensitivity, or certain medical conditions should exercise caution and consult with a healthcare provider before using bladderwrack supplements. Common side effects may include digestive upset, allergic reactions, or interactions with medications.

Blood Purifier:

Definition: Blood purifiers are herbal remedies or dietary supplements believed to cleanse or detoxify the blood, often promoting overall health and well-being. They are thought to support the body's natural detoxification processes and improve blood circulation.

Ingredients: Blood purifiers may contain a variety of herbs and botanical extracts known for their purported cleansing and detoxifying properties. Common ingredients include burdock root, red clover, dandelion root, and yellow dock root, among others.

How to Prepare: Blood purifiers are typically available in various forms, including capsules, tablets, powders, and liquid extracts. They are usually taken orally with water or juice, following the recommended dosage on the product label.

Dosage: The dosage of blood purifiers can vary depending on the specific product and individual needs. It's important to adhere to the recommended dosage on the product label or consult with a healthcare professional for personalized guidance.

How to Use: Blood purifiers are typically taken orally, either with water or mixed into beverages. They are often used as part of a detoxification regimen or to support overall health and vitality.

Side Effects: While blood purifiers are generally considered safe for most people when used as directed, some individuals may experience side effects such as digestive discomfort, allergic reactions, or interactions with medications. It's important to consult with a healthcare provider before starting any new supplement regimen, especially if you have underlying health conditions or are taking medications.

THE END